Thyroid Mastery

Your Complete Guide to Optimal Health and Wellness

by

DR. George Samuel

CONTENTS

Frequently Asked Questions

Q1. What is the thyroid gland, and what does it do?

- The thyroid gland is a small, butterfly-shaped gland located in the neck. It produces hormones (T3 and T4) that regulate metabolism, growth, and development.

Q2. What is hypothyroidism?

- Hypothyroidism is a condition where the thyroid gland does not produce enough thyroid hormones. This can lead to symptoms such as fatigue, weight gain, and cold intolerance.

Q3. What causes hypothyroidism?

- The most common cause of hypothyroidism is Hashimoto's thyroiditis, an autoimmune condition where the immune system attacks the thyroid gland. Other causes include thyroid surgery, radiation therapy, and certain medications.

Q4. What are the symptoms of hyperthyroidism?

- Hyperthyroidism is a condition where the thyroid gland produces too much thyroid hormone. Symptoms can include weight loss, rapid heartbeat, anxiety, and heat intolerance.

Q5. What causes hyperthyroidism?

- The most common cause of hyperthyroidism is Graves' disease, an autoimmune condition where the immune system stimulates the thyroid gland to produce excess hormones. Other causes include thyroid nodules and thyroiditis.

Q6. What are thyroid nodules, and are they cancerous?

- Thyroid nodules are lumps that form in the thyroid gland. Most thyroid nodules are noncancerous (benign), but some can be cancerous. Imaging tests and biopsies are used to determine if a nodule is cancerous.

Q7. What is thyroid cancer?

- Thyroid cancer is a type of cancer that starts in the cells of the thyroid gland. It is often detected as a lump in the neck and is usually treatable with surgery, radioactive iodine therapy, and sometimes radiation therapy or chemotherapy.

Q8. How is thyroid cancer diagnosed?

- Thyroid cancer is diagnosed through a combination of imaging tests (ultrasound, CT scan, MRI) and a biopsy (fine-needle aspiration) to examine the cells in the thyroid nodule for cancerous changes.

Q9. What is thyroiditis?

- Thyroiditis is inflammation of the thyroid gland. There are several types, including Hashimoto's thyroiditis (chronic autoimmune thyroiditis), subacute thyroiditis (viral infection), and postpartum thyroiditis (after childbirth).

Q10. Can thyroid disorders affect pregnancy?

- Yes, thyroid disorders can affect pregnancy. Untreated hypothyroidism or hyperthyroidism can lead to complications such as miscarriage, preterm birth, and developmental issues in the baby.

Q11. What is thyroid eye disease (Graves' ophthalmopathy)?

- Thyroid eye disease is a condition associated with Graves' disease, where the immune system attacks the tissues around the eyes. This can cause eye bulging, double vision, and eye pain.

Q12. How is thyroid eye disease treated?

- Treatment for thyroid eye disease may include medications to reduce inflammation, steroids, orbital decompression surgery, and radiation therapy.

Q13. Is there a special diet for thyroid health?

- While there is no specific diet for thyroid health, eating a balanced diet rich in fruits, vegetables, lean proteins, and whole grains can support overall health, including thyroid function.

Q14. Can I take supplements for thyroid health?

- Some supplements, such as iodine, selenium, and vitamin D, may support thyroid function. However, it's important to talk to your healthcare provider before taking any supplements, as they can interact with medications and affect thyroid hormone levels.

Q15. Can stress affect thyroid function?

- Yes, chronic stress can affect thyroid function. Stress hormones can interfere with the production and regulation of thyroid hormones, leading to imbalances.

Q16. What is the treatment for hypothyroidism?

- The most common treatment for hypothyroidism is levothyroxine, a synthetic thyroid hormone replacement. It is taken orally to replace the missing thyroid hormone.

Q17. What is the treatment for hyperthyroidism?

- Treatment for hyperthyroidism may include antithyroid medications (such as methimazole or propylthiouracil), radioactive iodine therapy, or surgery to remove part or all of the thyroid gland.

Q18. Can thyroid disorders cause hair loss?

- Yes, thyroid disorders can cause hair loss. Both hypothyroidism and hyperthyroidism can disrupt the normal cycle of hair growth, leading to hair thinning or loss.

Q19. Can thyroid disorders cause weight gain?

- Hypothyroidism can lead to weight gain due to a slowed metabolism, while hyperthyroidism can cause weight loss due to an increased metabolism. However, weight gain or loss can also be influenced by other factors, so it's important to consult with a healthcare provider for an accurate diagnosis.

Q20. Can thyroid disorders be cured?

- In some cases, thyroid disorders can be effectively managed with medication or other treatments. However, certain conditions, such as autoimmune thyroiditis or thyroid cancer, may require ongoing management and monitoring.

Introduction

The Vital Role of the Thyroid Gland in Metabolism and Overall Health

The thyroid gland, a small but mighty organ located in the front of the neck, plays a crucial role in maintaining the body's metabolic balance and overall well-being. Despite its modest size, the thyroid gland exerts powerful effects on numerous bodily functions, influencing everything from heart rate and body temperature to energy levels and mood.

At the heart of the thyroid's function are the hormones it produces: thyroxine (T4) and triiodothyronine (T3). These hormones are synthesized from iodine, an essential mineral found in certain foods and supplements. The production of T4 and T3 is tightly regulated by the hypothalamus and pituitary gland in a feedback loop known as the hypothalamic-pituitary-thyroid (HPT) axis.

The thyroid hormones T4 and T3 play a pivotal role in regulating metabolism, which is the process by which the body converts food into energy. They do this by influencing the rate at which cells use oxygen and produce heat, thereby affecting the body's basal metabolic rate (BMR). A properly functioning thyroid gland helps maintain a healthy BMR, which is crucial for weight management and overall energy levels.

In addition to metabolism, thyroid hormones also impact other vital functions. They play a role in growth and development, particularly during infancy and childhood, influencing bone growth, brain development, and overall physical growth. Thyroid hormones are also essential for maintaining normal heart rate and rhythm, as well as for the proper functioning of the digestive system and reproductive system.

The thyroid gland's influence extends beyond physical health to mental and emotional well-being. Thyroid hormones can affect mood, cognition, and emotional stability. Imbalances in thyroid function can lead to symptoms such as depression, anxiety, and cognitive impairment.

Given the thyroid gland's central role in so many bodily functions, it is clear why maintaining its health is crucial for overall well-being. Understanding the thyroid gland's functions and how they impact the body is key to recognizing and managing thyroid disorders effectively. Throughout this book, we will explore the various thyroid disorders, their causes, symptoms, diagnosis, and treatment options, empowering you with the knowledge to take charge of your thyroid health.

Overview of the book's purpose and structure

Welcome to "Thyroid Mastery: Your Complete Guide to Optimal Health and Wellness" This book is designed to provide you with comprehensive information about the thyroid gland, its functions, common disorders, diagnosis, treatment options, and tips for maintaining thyroid health. Whether you're newly diagnosed with a thyroid condition, have been managing one for years, or simply want to learn more about this vital gland and its impact on your health, this book aims to be your go-to resource.

Purpose of the Book

The primary purpose of this book is to empower you with knowledge and understanding of thyroid health. We aim to demystify complex medical concepts related to the thyroid gland and its disorders, making them accessible and easy to comprehend. By gaining a deeper understanding of how the thyroid works and the various conditions that can affect it, you'll be better equipped to make informed decisions about your health and work effectively with your healthcare team.

Structure of the Book

This book is organized into several chapters, each focusing on different aspects of thyroid health and related disorders. Here's a brief overview of what you can expect from each chapter:

- Chapter 1: Anatomy and Function of the Thyroid Gland provides a detailed look at the structure of the thyroid gland and its role in regulating metabolism, growth, and development.

- Chapter 2: Thyroid Disorders Overview offers an overview of the most common thyroid disorders, including hypothyroidism, hyperthyroidism, thyroid nodules, and thyroid cancer. You'll learn about their symptoms, causes, and risk factors.

- Chapter 3: Hypothyroidism delves into the details of this condition, covering its causes, symptoms, diagnosis, and treatment options, with a focus on levothyroxine therapy.

- Chapter 4: Hyperthyroidism explores the causes, symptoms, diagnosis, and treatment options for hyperthyroidism, including antithyroid medications, radioactive iodine therapy, and surgery.

- Chapter 5: Thyroid Nodules discusses the nature of thyroid nodules, how they are evaluated and diagnosed, and the various treatment options available.

- Chapter 6: Thyroid Cancer provides an in-depth look at different types of thyroid cancer, their causes, diagnosis, and treatment modalities, including surgery, radioactive iodine therapy, and targeted therapy.

- Chapter 7: Thyroiditis covers the different types of thyroiditis, their causes, symptoms, and treatment approaches, including medications and hormone replacement therapy.

- Chapter 8: Thyroid and Pregnancy explores the importance of thyroid function during pregnancy, its effects on pregnancy outcomes, and strategies for managing thyroid disorders during pregnancy.

- Chapter 9: Thyroid Eye Disease (Graves' Ophthalmopathy) focuses on the causes, symptoms, and treatment options for this condition, which is often associated with Graves' disease.

- Chapter 10: Thyroid Diet and Lifestyle offers practical tips for maintaining a healthy diet and lifestyle to support thyroid health, including the importance of nutrition, exercise, stress management, and sleep.

- Appendix: Thyroid Function Tests and Reference Ranges provides a handy reference for understanding common thyroid function tests and their interpretation. It also gives a clear and step by step approach to different stress management techniques.

- Glossary contains definitions of key terms related to thyroid health, ensuring that you can easily understand and navigate the content of this book.

We hope that this book will serve as a valuable resource on your journey to better understand and manage your thyroid health. By arming yourself with knowledge, you can take proactive steps towards optimal thyroid function and overall well-being.

Chapter 1

Anatomy and Function of the Thyroid Gland

Anatomy of the gland

The thyroid gland is a small, butterfly-shaped gland located in the front of the neck, just below the Adam's apple. Despite its small size, the thyroid plays a crucial role in regulating various bodily functions through the hormones it produces.

Anatomy of the Thyroid Gland

- Location: The thyroid gland is situated in the anterior neck, wrapped around the trachea (windpipe) just below the larynx (voice box).
- Structure: It consists of two lobes connected by a narrow band of tissue called the isthmus. Each lobe is roughly the size of a small plum and is shaped like a butterfly's wings, with the isthmus resembling the body of the butterfly.
- Blood Supply: The thyroid gland receives its blood supply from the superior thyroid artery, which

branches off from the external carotid artery, and the inferior thyroid artery, which branches off from the thyrocervical trunk.
- Nerve Supply: Nerve fibers from the sympathetic and parasympathetic nervous systems provide innervation to the thyroid gland, regulating its function.

Function of the Thyroid Gland

The main function of the thyroid gland is to produce hormones that regulate metabolism, growth, and development. The two primary hormones produced by the thyroid gland are thyroxine (T4) and triiodothyronine (T3), along with a small amount of calcitonin.

The production of thyroid hormones is regulated by the hypothalamus and pituitary gland through a feedback mechanism. The hypothalamus releases thyrotropin-releasing hormone (TRH), which stimulates the pituitary gland to produce thyroid-stimulating hormone (TSH). TSH then stimulates the thyroid gland to produce and release T3 and T4 into the bloodstream. As the levels of T3 and T4 increase, they inhibit the release of TRH and TSH, creating a feedback loop that helps maintain thyroid hormone levels within a narrow range.

Hormones produced by the thyroid (T3, T4, calcitonin) and their functions

The thyroid gland is a crucial part of the endocrine system, responsible for producing hormones that play vital roles in regulating metabolism, growth, and development. Understanding the anatomy and function of the thyroid gland is fundamental to grasping how thyroid disorders can impact overall health.

- Triiodothyronine (T3): T3 is the more active form of thyroid hormone, responsible for regulating metabolism, body temperature, and heart rate. It plays a crucial role in the body's energy production and utilization.

- Thyroxine (T4): T4 is the precursor to T3 and is produced in larger quantities by the thyroid gland. It is converted into T3 in various tissues throughout the body. T4 also plays a role in regulating metabolism and energy levels.

- Calcitonin: Calcitonin is involved in regulating calcium levels in the blood. It works in opposition to parathyroid hormone (PTH) to help maintain calcium balance in the body by promoting calcium deposition in bones and inhibiting calcium reabsorption in the kidneys.

Functions of Thyroid Hormones

The hormones produced by the thyroid gland have several important functions:

- Regulating Metabolism: T3 and T4 play a crucial role in regulating the body's metabolism, which is the process of converting food into energy. They help control how quickly the body burns calories and uses energy.

- Growth and Development: Thyroid hormones are essential for normal growth and development, especially in children. They help regulate the growth of bones, muscles, and other tissues.

- Body Temperature Regulation: Thyroid hormones influence the body's temperature regulation mechanisms. They can affect how the body responds to changes in temperature and help maintain a stable internal body temperature.

- Heart Rate and Blood Pressure: Thyroid hormones influence heart rate and blood pressure. They can affect the rate at which the heart beats and how forcefully it contracts, which can impact blood pressure.

Role of the thyroid in metabolism, growth, and development

1. Regulation of Metabolism: The thyroid hormones T3 and T4 play a key role in regulating the body's metabolism, which is the process by which the body converts food into energy. These hormones influence the rate at which cells use oxygen and produce heat and energy from nutrients.

2. Growth and Development: Thyroid hormones are critical for normal growth and development, particularly in infants and children. They help regulate the growth of tissues and organs, including the brain, bones, and muscles. Thyroid hormones also play a role in the development of the nervous system and the maturation of reproductive organs.

3. Regulation of Body Temperature: Thyroid hormones help regulate body temperature by influencing the rate of heat production and heat loss in the body. They can affect how quickly the body burns calories and generates heat, which is important for maintaining a stable body temperature.

4. Heart Rate and Blood Pressure: Thyroid hormones can influence heart rate and blood pressure by affecting the sensitivity of blood vessels to certain hormones and the responsiveness of the heart to signals from the nervous system.

5. Metabolic Rate: The thyroid gland helps regulate the body's metabolic rate, which is the rate at which the body burns calories to produce energy. This can affect weight management and overall energy levels.

Chapter 2

Thyroid Disorders Overview

Common thyroid disorders: hypothyroidism, hyperthyroidism, thyroid nodules, thyroid cancer

Thyroid disorders are conditions that affect the function and structure of the thyroid gland, leading to various symptoms and health implications. Understanding these disorders is crucial for proper diagnosis, treatment, and management. Here, we will explore four common thyroid disorders: hypothyroidism, hyperthyroidism, thyroid nodules, and thyroid cancer.

1. Hypothyroidism

Definition: Hypothyroidism occurs when the thyroid gland does not produce enough thyroid hormones, primarily thyroxine (T4) and triiodothyronine (T3). This can slow down the body's metabolism and lead to a range of symptoms, including fatigue, weight gain, cold intolerance, dry skin, and hair loss.

Causes: The most common cause of hypothyroidism is Hashimoto's thyroiditis, an autoimmune condition where the immune system attacks the thyroid gland. Other causes include thyroid surgery, radiation therapy, certain medications (e.g., lithium, amiodarone), and congenital thyroid abnormalities.

Diagnosis: Hypothyroidism is diagnosed through blood tests that measure levels of thyroid-stimulating hormone (TSH) and thyroid hormones (T4 and T3). High TSH levels with low T4 levels indicate hypothyroidism.

Treatment: The standard treatment for hypothyroidism is levothyroxine, a synthetic form of T4 hormone, taken orally to replace the missing hormone. Regular monitoring of thyroid hormone levels is necessary to adjust the dosage as needed.

2. Hyperthyroidism

Definition: Hyperthyroidism is the opposite of hypothyroidism, characterized by an overactive thyroid gland that produces excessive thyroid hormones. This can lead to symptoms such as weight loss, rapid heartbeat, anxiety, tremors, and heat intolerance.

Causes: The most common cause of hyperthyroidism is Graves' disease, an autoimmune condition where the immune system mistakenly stimulates the thyroid gland to produce excess hormones. Other causes include toxic nodular goiter (enlarged thyroid with nodules producing excess hormones) and thyroiditis (inflammation of the thyroid gland).

Diagnosis: Hyperthyroidism is diagnosed through blood tests that measure TSH, T4, and T3 levels. Low TSH levels with high T4 and T3 levels indicate hyperthyroidism.

Treatment: Treatment options for hyperthyroidism include antithyroid medications (e.g., methimazole, propylthiouracil) to reduce hormone production, radioactive iodine therapy to destroy part of the thyroid gland, or surgery to remove part or all of the thyroid gland.

3. Thyroid Nodules

Definition: Thyroid nodules are lumps or growths that form within the thyroid gland. Most nodules are benign (noncancerous) and do not cause symptoms. However, some nodules can be cancerous or cause symptoms such as difficulty swallowing, hoarseness, or neck discomfort.

Causes: The exact cause of thyroid nodules is often unknown. Factors that may contribute to their development include iodine deficiency, inflammation of the thyroid gland, genetic predisposition, and radiation exposure.

Diagnosis: Thyroid nodules are typically detected during a physical examination or imaging tests (e.g., ultrasound, CT scan). A fine-needle aspiration biopsy may be performed to determine if a nodule is cancerous.

Treatment: Treatment for thyroid nodules depends on their size, appearance, and whether they are causing symptoms. Options include observation (if the nodule is small and noncancerous), thyroid hormone suppression therapy, radioactive iodine therapy, or surgery to remove the nodule.

4. Thyroid Cancer

Definition: Thyroid cancer is a type of cancer that develops in the cells of the thyroid gland. It is relatively rare but is often curable if detected early. The most common types of thyroid cancer are papillary carcinoma, follicular carcinoma, medullary carcinoma, and anaplastic carcinoma.

Causes: The exact cause of thyroid cancer is not fully understood. However, risk factors include a family history of thyroid cancer, radiation exposure (especially during childhood), certain genetic syndromes (e.g., multiple endocrine neoplasia type 2), and iodine deficiency.

Diagnosis: Thyroid cancer is diagnosed through a combination of imaging tests (e.g., ultrasound, CT scan, MRI) and a biopsy (fine-needle aspiration) to examine the cells for cancerous changes.

Treatment: Treatment for thyroid cancer depends on the type and stage of the cancer. It may include surgery to remove part or all of the thyroid gland (thyroidectomy), radioactive iodine therapy to destroy remaining thyroid tissue, targeted therapy, radiation therapy, or hormone replacement therapy.

Importance of thyroid function tests for diagnosis

Thyroid function tests are essential tools used by healthcare providers to assess the health of the thyroid gland and diagnose thyroid disorders. These tests measure the levels of thyroid hormones (T3 and T4) and thyroid-stimulating hormone (TSH) in the blood, providing valuable insights into the functioning of the thyroid gland.

1. TSH Test: Thyroid-stimulating hormone (TSH) is produced by the pituitary gland and plays a crucial role in regulating the thyroid gland's hormone production. When the thyroid gland is not producing enough hormones (hypothyroidism), the pituitary gland increases its production of TSH to stimulate the thyroid gland. Conversely, when the thyroid gland is overactive (hyperthyroidism), the pituitary gland reduces its production of TSH. A high TSH level indicates hypothyroidism, while a low TSH level indicates hyperthyroidism.

2. T3 and T4 Tests: These tests measure the levels of triiodothyronine (T3) and thyroxine (T4), which are the two main thyroid hormones. T4 is the primary hormone produced by the thyroid gland, and most of it is converted into T3, the more active form of the hormone. Low levels of T3 and T4 indicate hypothyroidism, while high levels indicate hyperthyroidism.

3. Thyroid Antibody Tests: These tests measure the levels of antibodies that the immune system produces against the thyroid gland. Elevated levels of thyroid antibodies are indicative of autoimmune thyroid disorders, such as Hashimoto's thyroiditis (associated with hypothyroidism) or Graves' disease (associated with hyperthyroidism).

4. Thyroid Ultrasound: In addition to blood tests, a thyroid ultrasound may be performed to assess the size, shape, and texture of the thyroid gland. This imaging test can help identify thyroid nodules, inflammation, or other structural abnormalities that may require further evaluation.

5. Fine-Needle Aspiration Biopsy: If a thyroid nodule is found during an ultrasound, a fine-needle aspiration

biopsy may be recommended to determine if the nodule is benign or cancerous. During this procedure, a small sample of tissue is extracted from the nodule and examined under a microscope.

Chapter 3: Hypothyroidism

Hypothyroidism is a common thyroid disorder characterized by an underactive thyroid gland, which fails to produce enough thyroid hormones (T3 and T4) to meet the body's needs. This can lead to a wide range of symptoms and health issues, affecting various systems in the body. Understanding the definition, causes, and risk factors of hypothyroidism is essential for recognizing and managing this condition effectively.

Definition of Hypothyroidism

Hypothyroidism occurs when the thyroid gland does not produce sufficient thyroid hormones to maintain normal bodily functions. This can lead to a slowdown in metabolism, affecting many aspects of health, including energy levels, weight management, and overall well-being. The condition can develop slowly over time, and symptoms may be subtle and easily overlooked initially.

Causes of Hypothyroidism

1. Autoimmune Thyroiditis (Hashimoto's Thyroiditis): This is the most common cause of hypothyroidism in developed countries. It occurs when the body's immune system mistakenly attacks the thyroid gland, leading to inflammation and eventual destruction of thyroid tissue. This autoimmune reaction impairs the gland's ability to produce thyroid hormones.

2. Thyroid Surgery or Radiation Therapy: Surgical removal of all or part of the thyroid gland (thyroidectomy) or radiation therapy to the neck area can damage the thyroid gland, leading to hypothyroidism. This is more common in individuals treated for thyroid cancer or other thyroid conditions.

3. Iodine Deficiency: Iodine is an essential mineral required for the production of thyroid hormones. In areas where iodine deficiency is prevalent, such as certain parts of the world with low dietary iodine intake, hypothyroidism can occur. However, iodine deficiency is rare in developed countries due to iodized salt and other dietary sources of iodine.

4. Medications: Certain medications, such as lithium (used to treat bipolar disorder), amiodarone (used to treat heart rhythm problems), and some anti-thyroid medications, can interfere with thyroid hormone production and lead to hypothyroidism.

5. Congenital Hypothyroidism: Some babies are born with an underactive thyroid gland, either due to a developmental defect or an inherited condition. This is known as congenital hypothyroidism and requires prompt treatment to prevent developmental delays and other complications.

6. Pituitary or Hypothalamic Disorders: In rare cases, hypothyroidism can result from disorders affecting the pituitary gland or hypothalamus, which are involved in regulating thyroid hormone production. These conditions can disrupt the release of thyroid-stimulating hormone (TSH), which is necessary for stimulating the thyroid gland.

Risk Factors for Hypothyroidism

- Age: Hypothyroidism can occur at any age, but it is more common in older adults, particularly women over the age of 60.

- Gender: Women are more likely to develop hypothyroidism than men, especially after childbirth or menopause.
- Family History: Having a family history of thyroid disorders, particularly autoimmune thyroiditis, increases the risk of developing hypothyroidism.
- Iodine Intake: Inadequate dietary iodine intake can increase the risk of hypothyroidism, although this is rare in areas with iodized salt.
- Previous Thyroid Surgery or Radiation Therapy: Individuals who have undergone thyroid surgery or radiation therapy to the neck area are at higher risk of developing hypothyroidism.
- Certain Medications: Long-term use of medications that can interfere with thyroid function, such as lithium or amiodarone, can increase the risk of hypothyroidism.

Signs and Symptoms

1. Fatigue: One of the hallmark symptoms of hypothyroidism is persistent fatigue or feeling tired despite getting enough sleep. This fatigue may be debilitating and can significantly impact daily activities and quality of life.

2. Weight Gain: Hypothyroidism can lead to unexplained weight gain or difficulty losing weight, even with diet and exercise. This is due to a slowed metabolism, which can cause the body to burn calories at a slower rate than usual.

3. Cold Intolerance: People with hypothyroidism often feel cold, especially in their hands and feet, even in warm environments. This intolerance to cold is related to the thyroid hormone's role in regulating body temperature.

4. Depression: Hypothyroidism can affect mood and lead to feelings of depression or low mood. This may be accompanied by other symptoms of depression, such as sadness, loss of interest in activities, and changes in appetite or sleep patterns.

5. Dry Skin and Hair: The lack of thyroid hormones can lead to dry, rough, and pale skin, as well as brittle hair that may fall out more easily. Nails may also become brittle and prone to splitting.

6. Constipation: Hypothyroidism can slow down the digestive system, leading to constipation. This is due

to reduced movement of the intestines, which can result in hard, dry stools that are difficult to pass.

7. Muscle Weakness and Joint Pain: Some people with hypothyroidism may experience muscle weakness, aches, and stiffness, particularly in the arms and legs. Joint pain and stiffness, especially in the hands and feet, are also common.

8. Memory Problems and Brain Fog: Hypothyroidism can affect cognitive function, leading to memory problems, difficulty concentrating, and a feeling of mental fog or confusion.

9. Irregular Menstrual Periods: In women, hypothyroidism can lead to irregular menstrual periods, including heavier or lighter bleeding than usual, or skipped periods.

10. Hoarse Voice: A hoarse or raspy voice can be a symptom of hypothyroidism, as the thyroid gland's enlargement (goiter) can press on the vocal cords and affect voice quality.

Diagnosis of Hypothyroidism

Diagnosing hypothyroidism involves a combination of clinical evaluation, thyroid function tests, and sometimes additional imaging or antibody tests. The primary diagnostic tools include:

1. Thyroid Function Tests: Blood tests are used to measure levels of thyroid-stimulating hormone (TSH), thyroxine (T4), and triiodothyronine (T3). In hypothyroidism, TSH levels are typically elevated, indicating that the thyroid gland is not producing enough hormones. T4 levels may also be low, confirming the diagnosis.

2. Clinical Evaluation: Your healthcare provider will assess your symptoms, medical history, and physical examination findings. Common symptoms of hypothyroidism include fatigue, weight gain, cold intolerance, dry skin, and hair loss.

3. Thyroid Antibody Tests: In cases where autoimmune thyroiditis (such as Hashimoto's thyroiditis) is suspected, antibody tests may be performed to check for elevated levels of thyroid peroxidase antibodies (TPOAb) or thyroglobulin antibodies (TgAb). These antibodies are indicative of autoimmune thyroid disease.

4. Thyroid Ultrasound: In some cases, a thyroid ultrasound may be recommended to assess the size, shape, and texture of the thyroid gland and to identify any nodules or abnormalities.

Treatment of Hypothyroidism

The mainstay of treatment for hypothyroidism is hormone replacement therapy with levothyroxine, a synthetic form of thyroxine (T4). This medication is taken orally and works to restore thyroid hormone levels to normal. Key aspects of treatment include:

1. Levothyroxine Therapy: The goal of levothyroxine therapy is to normalize thyroid hormone levels in the body. The dosage is typically started at a low level and gradually increased based on blood tests and symptoms. It's important to take levothyroxine consistently and as prescribed by your healthcare provider.

2. Monitoring: Regular monitoring of thyroid function tests is essential to ensure that the dosage of levothyroxine is appropriate. Blood tests are usually

repeated 6-8 weeks after starting or adjusting the medication, and then annually once stable.

3. Dietary Considerations: While there is no specific diet for hypothyroidism, some dietary considerations may be helpful. Eating a balanced diet with sufficient iodine, selenium, and other nutrients is important for overall thyroid health. However, excessive iodine intake should be avoided, especially in cases of autoimmune thyroiditis.

4. Lifestyle Modifications: Maintaining a healthy lifestyle with regular exercise, stress management, and adequate sleep can support overall thyroid health and may help manage symptoms of hypothyroidism.

5. Compliance: It's crucial to take levothyroxine as prescribed and not to skip doses or stop the medication without consulting your healthcare provider. Consistent adherence to treatment is key to effectively managing hypothyroidism.

6. Potential Interactions: Some medications, supplements, and dietary factors can interfere with the absorption or effectiveness of levothyroxine. It's important to discuss all medications and supplements

with your healthcare provider to avoid potential interactions.

Chapter 4: Hyperthyroidism

Hyperthyroidism is a condition characterized by an overactive thyroid gland that produces an excess of thyroid hormones, primarily thyroxine (T4) and triiodothyronine (T3). These hormones play a key role in regulating metabolism, and an excess can lead to a wide range of symptoms and complications.

Causes of Hyperthyroidism

1. Graves' Disease: The most common cause of hyperthyroidism is Graves' disease, an autoimmune disorder where the immune system produces antibodies that stimulate the thyroid gland to produce too much thyroid hormone. This condition is often associated with other autoimmune disorders.

2. Thyroid Nodules: Hyperthyroidism can also be caused by nodules in the thyroid gland that produce excess thyroid hormone independently of the normal regulatory mechanisms. These nodules can be benign (noncancerous) or malignant (cancerous).

3. Thyroiditis: Inflammation of the thyroid gland, known as thyroiditis, can cause a temporary increase in thyroid hormone levels. This can occur with subacute thyroiditis (viral infection), postpartum thyroiditis (after childbirth), or silent thyroiditis (unknown cause).

4. Excessive Iodine Intake: Consuming too much iodine, either through diet or medication, can lead to hyperthyroidism, especially in individuals with underlying thyroid disorders or iodine sensitivity.

5. Medications: Certain medications, such as amiodarone (used to treat heart rhythm disorders), can contain high levels of iodine and can induce hyperthyroidism in susceptible individuals.

6. Other Causes: Less common causes of hyperthyroidism include thyroid cancer, pituitary gland disorders, and rare tumors that produce thyroid-like hormones.

Risk Factors for Hyperthyroidism

Several factors may increase the risk of developing hyperthyroidism, including:

- Gender: Women are more likely than men to develop hyperthyroidism, especially during their childbearing years and menopause.
- Age: Hyperthyroidism can occur at any age but is more common in individuals over 60 years old.
- Family History: A family history of thyroid disorders, particularly Graves' disease, increases the risk of developing hyperthyroidism.
- Autoimmune Disorders: Having other autoimmune disorders, such as type 1 diabetes or rheumatoid arthritis, can increase the risk of autoimmune thyroid conditions like Graves' disease.
- Pregnancy: Pregnancy and the postpartum period can increase the risk of developing postpartum thyroiditis, a form of hyperthyroidism that occurs after childbirth.

Signs and Symptoms of Hyperthyroidism

1. Weight Loss: Unexplained weight loss despite increased appetite is a common symptom of hyperthyroidism. This occurs due to an accelerated metabolism, which leads to increased calorie burning

and weight loss, even with a normal or increased food intake.

2. Rapid Heartbeat (Tachycardia): Hyperthyroidism can cause the heart to beat faster than normal, leading to palpitations, a feeling of rapid or irregular heartbeats, and potentially increased blood pressure. This occurs because thyroid hormones stimulate the heart to pump more blood at a faster rate.

3. Anxiety and Nervousness: Excessive thyroid hormone levels can affect the nervous system, leading to feelings of anxiety, nervousness, restlessness, and irritability. Patients may also experience difficulty concentrating and emotional instability.

4. Heat Intolerance and Sweating: Hyperthyroidism can increase the body's sensitivity to heat, leading to excessive sweating, even in cool environments. Patients may feel hot or flushed and have an increased need to cool down.

5. Fatigue and Weakness: Despite increased metabolism, some patients with hyperthyroidism may experience fatigue and weakness. This can be due to muscle weakness, decreased muscle mass, and overall

strain on the body from the increased metabolic activity.

6. Tremors and Shaking Hands: Hyperthyroidism can cause fine tremors, especially in the hands and fingers. These tremors are usually more pronounced during physical activity or when holding objects.

7. Increased Appetite: While weight loss is a common symptom, hyperthyroidism can also lead to an increased appetite, as the body's increased metabolic rate requires more energy intake.

8. Changes in Menstrual Patterns: Women with hyperthyroidism may experience irregular menstrual periods or even cessation of periods (amenorrhea). This can be due to hormonal imbalances caused by thyroid hormone excess.

9. Exophthalmos (Bulging Eyes): In Graves' disease, a common cause of hyperthyroidism, some patients develop a condition known as exophthalmos, where the eyes appear to bulge out of their sockets. This is due to inflammation and swelling of the tissues behind the eyes.

10. Other Symptoms: Other less common symptoms of hyperthyroidism include hair loss, brittle nails, thinning of the skin, increased bowel movements or diarrhea, and difficulty sleeping.

Diagnosis of Hyperthyroidism

Diagnosing hyperthyroidism involves a thorough evaluation of symptoms, physical examination findings, and thyroid function tests. Key steps in the diagnostic process include:

1. Thyroid Function Tests: Blood tests are used to measure levels of thyroid hormones, including thyroxine (T4) and triiodothyronine (T3), as well as thyroid-stimulating hormone (TSH). In hyperthyroidism, T4 and T3 levels are typically elevated, while TSH levels are suppressed.

2. Clinical Evaluation: Your healthcare provider will assess your symptoms, medical history, and physical examination findings. Common symptoms of hyperthyroidism include weight loss, rapid or irregular heartbeat, anxiety, tremors, and heat intolerance.

3. Thyroid Antibody Tests: In cases where autoimmune hyperthyroidism (such as Graves' disease) is suspected, antibody tests may be performed to check for elevated levels of thyroid-stimulating immunoglobulins (TSI) or thyroid peroxidase antibodies (TPOAb). These antibodies are indicative of autoimmune thyroid disease.

4. Radioactive Iodine Uptake (RAIU) Test: This test measures the amount of radioactive iodine taken up by the thyroid gland. It can help determine the cause of hyperthyroidism and assess thyroid function.

5. Thyroid Ultrasound: In some cases, a thyroid ultrasound may be recommended to assess the size, shape, and texture of the thyroid gland and to identify any nodules or abnormalities.

Treatment of Hyperthyroidism

The treatment approach for hyperthyroidism depends on the underlying cause, severity of symptoms, and individual patient factors. Common treatment options include:

1. Antithyroid Medications: These medications, such as methimazole (Tapazole) or propylthiouracil (PTU), work by blocking the production of thyroid hormones. They are often used as a first-line treatment to control symptoms and normalize thyroid function. Treatment duration varies depending on the response and may last for several months to years.

2. Radioactive Iodine Therapy (RAI): This treatment involves the oral administration of radioactive iodine, which is taken up by the thyroid gland and destroys thyroid cells. RAI is a common treatment for Graves' disease and toxic nodular goiter. It is effective in reducing thyroid hormone levels but may lead to hypothyroidism over time, requiring lifelong thyroid hormone replacement therapy.

3. Thyroidectomy (Surgery): In cases where antithyroid medications and RAI are not suitable or effective, surgical removal of part or all of the thyroid gland (thyroidectomy) may be recommended. This approach is often used for large goiters, nodules suspicious for cancer, or when other treatments have failed or are contraindicated. Thyroidectomy may result in permanent hypothyroidism, requiring lifelong thyroid hormone replacement therapy.

4. Beta-Blockers: These medications, such as propranolol or atenolol, are used to manage symptoms of hyperthyroidism, such as rapid heartbeat, tremors, and anxiety. They do not treat the underlying cause but can provide symptomatic relief while other treatments take effect.

5. Monitoring: Regular monitoring of thyroid function tests is essential during treatment to assess the effectiveness of therapy and adjust treatment as needed. Blood tests are typically repeated every 4-8 weeks initially, then less frequently once stable.

6. Pregnancy Considerations: Treatment of hyperthyroidism during pregnancy requires special considerations to ensure the health of both the mother and the baby. It's important to work closely with a healthcare provider experienced in managing thyroid disorders during pregnancy.

Chapter 5: Thyroid Nodules

Definition of Thyroid Nodules

Thyroid nodules are abnormal growths or lumps that form within the thyroid gland. They can vary in size, shape, and composition, and they may be solitary or multiple. Most thyroid nodules are benign (non-cancerous) and do not cause any symptoms. However, in some cases, thyroid nodules can be malignant (cancerous) and require further evaluation and treatment.

Types of Thyroid Nodules

1. Benign Nodules: The majority of thyroid nodules are benign and are not associated with cancer. These nodules may be classified into various types based on their composition and appearance on imaging studies:
   - Colloid Nodules: Also known as follicular adenomas, these nodules are made up of thyroid follicles filled with colloid, a substance that stores thyroid hormones. Colloid nodules are usually benign

and do not require treatment unless they cause symptoms or grow significantly in size.

   - Cystic Nodules: These nodules contain fluid-filled cysts and may have a smooth, round appearance on ultrasound. Cystic nodules are typically benign but may require evaluation if they cause symptoms or if there are concerning features on imaging.

   - Mixed Nodules: These nodules have both solid and cystic components. They may be benign or malignant, depending on their characteristics and the presence of suspicious features.

2. Malignant Nodules: A small percentage of thyroid nodules are malignant, meaning they are cancerous. The most common type of thyroid cancer associated with nodules is papillary thyroid carcinoma, followed by follicular thyroid carcinoma. Other less common types include medullary thyroid carcinoma and anaplastic thyroid carcinoma. Malignant nodules require prompt evaluation and treatment to prevent the spread of cancer.

Risk Factors for Thyroid Nodules

Several factors may increase the risk of developing thyroid nodules, including:

1. Age and Gender: Thyroid nodules are more common in older adults and in women.
2. Family History: A family history of thyroid nodules or thyroid cancer can increase the risk.
3. Radiation Exposure: Previous exposure to radiation, especially during childhood or adolescence, increases the risk of developing thyroid nodules and thyroid cancer.
4. Iodine Deficiency or Excess: Both iodine deficiency and excess can contribute to the development of thyroid nodules. Iodine is essential for thyroid hormone production, and inadequate or excessive intake can disrupt thyroid function.
5. Thyroiditis: Chronic inflammation of the thyroid gland, such as Hashimoto's thyroiditis or chronic lymphocytic thyroiditis, may increase the risk of nodules.
6. Dietary Factors: Certain dietary factors, such as a diet low in iodine or high in goitrogens (substances that interfere with thyroid function), may play a role in the development of thyroid nodules.

Evaluation and Diagnosis of Thyroid Nodules

Thyroid nodules are common and often benign (non-cancerous), but they require careful evaluation to determine their nature and whether further investigation or treatment is needed. The evaluation of thyroid nodules typically involves a combination of imaging studies, such as ultrasound, and, in some cases, a fine-needle aspiration biopsy (FNAB). Here's a detailed look at these diagnostic approaches:

1. Thyroid Ultrasound: Ultrasound is the primary imaging modality used to evaluate thyroid nodules. It provides detailed information about the size, shape, texture, and vascularity (blood flow) of the nodules. Ultrasound can help distinguish between solid nodules (composed of thyroid tissue) and cystic nodules (fluid-filled sacs), as well as identify features suggestive of malignancy (cancer), such as irregular borders, microcalcifications, or increased vascularity.

   - Key Ultrasound Findings:
     - Size: The size of the nodule is an important factor in determining the risk of malignancy. Larger nodules (>1 cm) are generally considered higher risk and may warrant further evaluation.
     - Composition: Solid nodules are more concerning than cystic nodules. Mixed nodules (both solid and

cystic components) are also common and require careful assessment.

   - Echogenicity: The echogenicity (brightness) of the nodule compared to surrounding thyroid tissue can provide clues about its composition. Hypoechoic nodules (darker than surrounding tissue) are more suspicious for malignancy.

   - Margins: Well-defined margins are characteristic of benign nodules, while irregular or spiculated margins may indicate malignancy.

   - Calcifications: Microcalcifications within the nodule are associated with a higher risk of malignancy, especially if they are punctate (small, discrete) or coarse (larger, irregular).

2. Fine-Needle Aspiration Biopsy (FNAB): FNAB is a minimally invasive procedure used to obtain a sample of cells from a thyroid nodule for microscopic examination. It is performed using a thin needle guided by ultrasound imaging to ensure accurate placement. FNAB is indicated in the following scenarios:

   - Indeterminate or Suspicious Ultrasound Findings: If ultrasound features suggest a nodule is suspicious for malignancy or indeterminate (uncertain risk), FNAB can help clarify the diagnosis.

- Large or Growing Nodules: Nodules that are large (>1 cm) or rapidly growing may be biopsied to rule out malignancy.

- Persistent Nodules: Nodules that persist despite treatment or monitoring may require biopsy to assess for malignancy.

- Results and Interpretation: The cytology (cellular) analysis of the biopsy sample is classified into various categories based on the risk of malignancy, ranging from benign to suspicious for malignancy. The results help guide further management decisions, including the need for surgery or continued monitoring.

- Risks and Considerations: FNAB is generally safe and well-tolerated, but there is a small risk of bleeding or infection at the biopsy site. Rarely, the needle may puncture nearby structures, such as blood vessels or nerves, but this is uncommon when performed by experienced practitioners.

Treatment Options for Thyroid Nodules

The management of thyroid nodules depends on several factors, including the size of the nodule, whether it is benign or cancerous, the presence of symptoms, and the patient's overall health. Treatment options for thyroid nodules include:

1. Observation (Watchful Waiting): Many thyroid nodules are benign and do not require immediate treatment. In cases where the nodule is small, asymptomatic, and not growing rapidly, your healthcare provider may recommend a period of observation with regular follow-up visits and imaging studies to monitor for any changes. This approach is often used for nodules that are less than 1 cm in size and have a low risk of malignancy.

2. Thyroid Hormone Suppression Therapy: In some cases, especially when nodules are causing hyperthyroidism or are at risk of becoming malignant, your healthcare provider may prescribe thyroid hormone replacement therapy (levothyroxine) to suppress the production of thyroid-stimulating hormone (TSH), which can help reduce the size of the nodules. This approach is typically used for nodules associated with a condition called toxic multinodular goiter.

3. Radioactive Iodine Therapy (RAI): Radioactive iodine may be used to treat thyroid nodules that are causing hyperthyroidism or are suspected to be cancerous. The radioactive iodine is taken up by the thyroid tissue, including the nodules, and destroys the abnormal cells. This treatment is often used for nodules associated with hyperthyroidism or for thyroid cancer.

4. Thyroidectomy (Surgery): Surgical removal of part or all of the thyroid gland (thyroidectomy) may be recommended in certain cases, such as:

  - When a nodule is large and causing symptoms such as difficulty swallowing or breathing.
  - When a nodule is suspicious for thyroid cancer based on imaging studies or biopsy results.
  - When other treatments have failed or are not appropriate.

  Thyroidectomy may involve removing only the affected lobe (lobectomy) or the entire thyroid gland (total thyroidectomy). It can be performed using traditional open surgery or minimally invasive techniques such as endoscopic or robotic-assisted surgery.

5. Percutaneous Ethanol Injection Therapy (PEIT): This minimally invasive procedure involves injecting ethanol (alcohol) directly into the thyroid nodule under ultrasound guidance. The ethanol causes the nodule to shrink by damaging its cells. PEIT is typically used for benign cystic nodules or solid nodules that are not suitable for surgery.

6. Thermal Ablation Techniques: These techniques, including laser ablation, radiofrequency ablation, and microwave ablation, use heat to destroy thyroid nodules. They are minimally invasive and can be effective for shrinking nodules, particularly those that are causing symptoms or are at risk of malignancy.

Chapter 6: Thyroid Cancer

Types of Thyroid Cancer

Thyroid cancer is a relatively rare but treatable type of cancer that develops in the cells of the thyroid gland. There are several types of thyroid cancer, each with distinct characteristics and treatment approaches. The main types of thyroid cancer include:

1. Papillary Thyroid Cancer (PTC): Papillary thyroid cancer is the most common type, accounting for about 80% of all thyroid cancer cases. It usually grows slowly and tends to spread to nearby lymph nodes in the neck rather than to distant organs. PTC often presents as a painless lump in the neck and is more common in women than men. It has a high cure rate, especially when diagnosed and treated early.

2. Follicular Thyroid Cancer (FTC): Follicular thyroid cancer accounts for about 15% of thyroid cancer cases. It tends to spread to distant organs, such as the lungs or bones, more often than papillary thyroid cancer.

FTC may present as a nodule in the thyroid gland and is more common in older adults. Like PTC, FTC has a good prognosis with early detection and appropriate treatment.

3. Medullary Thyroid Cancer (MTC): Medullary thyroid cancer arises from the parafollicular cells (C cells) of the thyroid gland, which produce calcitonin. MTC accounts for about 3-5% of thyroid cancer cases. It can occur sporadically or be inherited as part of a genetic syndrome, such as multiple endocrine neoplasia type 2 (MEN2). MTC tends to grow more aggressively than papillary or follicular thyroid cancer and may spread to lymph nodes and distant organs. It requires specialized management, including genetic testing and surveillance for related syndromes.

4. Anaplastic Thyroid Cancer (ATC): Anaplastic thyroid cancer is the most aggressive and least common type of thyroid cancer, accounting for less than 2% of cases. It grows rapidly and is often diagnosed at an advanced stage when it has already spread to surrounding tissues and organs. ATC is challenging to treat and has a poor prognosis, with a low survival rate. Treatment usually involves a combination of surgery, radiation therapy, and chemotherapy.

In addition to these primary types, there are also variants and subtypes of thyroid cancer that may have distinct features and treatment considerations. These include variants of papillary and follicular thyroid cancer, such as tall cell variant, columnar cell variant, and oncocytic (Hürthle cell) variant, among others. Each subtype may have specific characteristics that influence its behavior and response to treatment.

Risk Factors and Causes of Thyroid Cancer

Thyroid cancer occurs when abnormal cells in the thyroid gland grow and divide uncontrollably, forming a tumor. While the exact cause of thyroid cancer is often unknown, several risk factors have been identified that may increase the likelihood of developing this condition. These include:

1. Gender: Thyroid cancer is more common in women than in men, with women being three times more likely to develop the disease. The reason for this gender difference is not fully understood, but it may be related to hormonal factors.

2. Age: Thyroid cancer can occur at any age, but it is most commonly diagnosed in people between the ages of 30 and 60. The risk increases with age, with the highest incidence in people over 60 years old.

3. Radiation Exposure: Exposure to high levels of radiation, especially during childhood, is a significant risk factor for thyroid cancer. This includes exposure from medical treatments (such as radiation therapy for head and neck cancers), environmental sources (such as nuclear accidents or fallout), or occupational exposure (such as working in nuclear power plants).

4. Family History: A family history of thyroid cancer or certain hereditary conditions, such as familial adenomatous polyposis (FAP) or multiple endocrine neoplasia type 2 (MEN2), can increase the risk of developing thyroid cancer. Genetic mutations associated with these conditions can predispose individuals to thyroid cancer.

5. Iodine Deficiency or Excess: Both iodine deficiency and excess can increase the risk of thyroid cancer, although the exact mechanism is not fully understood. Iodine is essential for thyroid hormone production, and inadequate or excessive iodine intake can affect

thyroid function and potentially contribute to the development of thyroid cancer.

6. Benign Thyroid Conditions: Certain benign thyroid conditions, such as goiter (enlarged thyroid gland) or thyroid nodules, may be associated with an increased risk of thyroid cancer, especially if the nodules are large or have certain characteristics (such as being solid rather than fluid-filled).

7. Dietary Factors: Some studies suggest that a diet low in fruits and vegetables and high in processed foods or red meat may be associated with an increased risk of thyroid cancer, although more research is needed to establish a clear link.

8. Obesity: Obesity has been identified as a potential risk factor for thyroid cancer, particularly the more aggressive forms of the disease. The exact mechanism underlying this association is not fully understood but may be related to hormonal and metabolic factors.

Diagnosis of Thyroid Cancer

The diagnosis of thyroid cancer involves a combination of clinical evaluation, imaging studies, biopsy, and thyroid function tests. Key steps in the diagnostic process include:

1. Imaging Studies: Ultrasound is often the first imaging test used to evaluate thyroid nodules and assess their characteristics, such as size, shape, and composition. Other imaging tests, such as computed tomography (CT) scans, magnetic resonance imaging (MRI), or positron emission tomography (PET) scans, may be performed to determine the extent of the cancer and whether it has spread to other parts of the body.

2. Fine-Needle Aspiration Biopsy (FNAB): This procedure involves using a thin needle to extract a sample of cells from the thyroid nodule for examination under a microscope. FNAB is the most reliable method for diagnosing thyroid cancer and determining the type of cancer present.

3. Thyroid Function Tests: Blood tests may be performed to assess thyroid hormone levels and thyroid function. While thyroid cancer itself does not usually affect thyroid hormone levels, these tests are important to evaluate overall thyroid function and guide treatment decisions.

4. Thyroid Antibody Tests: In cases where autoimmune thyroiditis (such as Hashimoto's thyroiditis) is suspected, antibody tests may be performed to check for elevated levels of thyroid peroxidase antibodies (TPOAb) or thyroglobulin antibodies (TgAb). These antibodies are indicative of autoimmune thyroid disease but are not specific for thyroid cancer.

Treatment Options for Thyroid Cancer

The treatment of thyroid cancer depends on the type and stage of the cancer, as well as the patient's overall health and preferences. Common treatment options include:

1. Surgery (Thyroidectomy): The primary treatment for thyroid cancer is surgical removal of part or all of the thyroid gland. The extent of surgery depends on the size and location of the cancer, as well as whether it has spread to nearby lymph nodes or other tissues. Types of thyroidectomy include:

  - Total Thyroidectomy: Removal of the entire thyroid gland.

- Partial Thyroidectomy (Lobectomy): Removal of one lobe of the thyroid gland, often used for smaller, localized cancers.

In some cases, additional lymph node dissection may be performed to remove cancerous lymph nodes in the neck.

2. Radioactive Iodine Therapy (RAI): After surgery, some patients may undergo RAI treatment to destroy any remaining thyroid tissue or cancer cells. Radioactive iodine is taken up by thyroid cells, including cancerous cells, and can help reduce the risk of recurrence. This treatment is often used for certain types of thyroid cancer, such as papillary and follicular thyroid cancer.

3. Thyroid Hormone Replacement Therapy: After surgery or RAI treatment, patients will need lifelong thyroid hormone replacement therapy with levothyroxine to maintain normal thyroid hormone levels. This medication replaces the hormones that the thyroid gland would normally produce and helps prevent hypothyroidism.

4. External Beam Radiation Therapy (EBRT): This treatment uses high-energy X-rays to kill cancer cells and shrink tumors. It is typically used in cases where the cancer has spread beyond the thyroid gland or has not responded to other treatments.

5. Targeted Therapy: In some cases, especially for advanced or metastatic thyroid cancer that does not respond to other treatments, targeted therapy drugs may be used. These medications target specific molecules involved in cancer growth and may help slow or stop the progression of the disease.

6. Chemotherapy: While chemotherapy is not commonly used for thyroid cancer, it may be considered in certain situations, such as when the cancer is aggressive or has spread to other parts of the body and is not responding to other treatments.

Chapter 7: Thyroiditis

Types of Thyroiditis

Thyroiditis refers to inflammation of the thyroid gland, which can result in a variety of symptoms and thyroid function abnormalities. There are several types of thyroiditis, each with its own causes, symptoms, and treatment approaches. The most common types include:

1. Hashimoto's Thyroiditis (Chronic Lymphocytic Thyroiditis): This is the most common cause of hypothyroidism in the United States. It is an autoimmune condition in which the immune system mistakenly attacks the thyroid gland, leading to inflammation and gradual destruction of thyroid tissue. Hashimoto's thyroiditis typically progresses slowly over years and can result in a gradual decline in thyroid function. Common symptoms include fatigue, weight gain, depression, dry skin, and sensitivity to cold. Treatment usually involves lifelong thyroid

hormone replacement therapy to restore normal thyroid hormone levels.

2. Postpartum Thyroiditis: This type of thyroiditis occurs in some women within the first year after giving birth. It is believed to be related to immune system changes that occur during pregnancy and the postpartum period. Postpartum thyroiditis can initially cause hyperthyroidism, followed by hypothyroidism, as the thyroid gland recovers. Symptoms can include fatigue, irritability, weight loss (during the hyperthyroid phase), and weight gain (during the hypothyroid phase). Most women recover normal thyroid function within 12-18 months, but some may develop permanent hypothyroidism requiring lifelong thyroid hormone replacement therapy.

3. Subacute Thyroiditis (De Quervain's Thyroiditis): This is a painful form of thyroiditis that typically follows a viral infection. It is thought to be caused by a viral infection that triggers an inflammatory response in the thyroid gland. Subacute thyroiditis can cause severe neck pain, fever, fatigue, and an enlarged, tender thyroid gland. It can also cause temporary hyperthyroidism due to the release of thyroid hormones from the inflamed gland. Treatment may

include nonsteroidal anti-inflammatory drugs (NSAIDs) for pain relief and, in some cases, beta-blockers to manage symptoms of hyperthyroidism. Most cases resolve within a few months, and thyroid function usually returns to normal, although some individuals may develop permanent hypothyroidism.

4. Silent (Painless) Thyroiditis: This type of thyroiditis is similar to postpartum thyroiditis but occurs in individuals who are not postpartum. It is characterized by inflammation of the thyroid gland without the typical symptoms of pain or tenderness. Silent thyroiditis can cause transient hyperthyroidism followed by hypothyroidism, similar to postpartum thyroiditis. The condition usually resolves on its own within a few months, but some individuals may develop permanent hypothyroidism.

5. Drug-Induced Thyroiditis: Some medications, such as amiodarone (used to treat heart rhythm disorders), interferon-alpha (used to treat certain cancers and viral infections), and lithium (used to treat bipolar disorder), can cause inflammation of the thyroid gland and disrupt thyroid function. The severity and duration of drug-induced thyroiditis can vary depending on the medication and individual response.

Treatment may involve discontinuing the offending medication or adjusting the dosage under the guidance of a healthcare provider.

6. Acute (Suppurative) Thyroiditis: This is a rare but serious form of thyroiditis caused by bacterial infection of the thyroid gland. It can lead to severe neck pain, fever, swelling, and difficulty swallowing or breathing. Acute thyroiditis requires prompt medical attention and treatment with antibiotics to resolve the infection. In some cases, drainage of pus from the infected gland may be necessary.

Treatment for thyroiditis depends on the underlying cause and severity of symptoms. In most cases, treatment focuses on managing symptoms and restoring normal thyroid function. This may include thyroid hormone replacement therapy for hypothyroidism, medications to control symptoms of hyperthyroidism, and pain management for inflammation-related discomfort. In some cases, anti-inflammatory medications or steroids may be prescribed to reduce inflammation in the thyroid gland.

Causes of Thyroiditis

Thyroiditis refers to inflammation of the thyroid gland, which can be caused by various factors, including:

1. Autoimmune Thyroiditis: The most common cause of thyroiditis is autoimmune thyroiditis, which includes Hashimoto's thyroiditis and atrophic thyroiditis. In these conditions, the immune system mistakenly attacks the thyroid gland, leading to inflammation and destruction of thyroid tissue. This can eventually result in hypothyroidism as the thyroid gland becomes unable to produce enough thyroid hormones.

2. Viral Infections: Viral infections, such as mumps, influenza, or Epstein-Barr virus, can sometimes trigger thyroiditis by causing inflammation of the thyroid gland. This is usually a temporary condition that resolves once the infection clears.

3. Bacterial Infections: In rare cases, bacterial infections can lead to thyroiditis, usually as a result of an infection spreading from nearby structures in the neck or from a systemic infection.

4. Drug-induced Thyroiditis: Certain medications, such as interferon-alpha, amiodarone, lithium, and cytokines, can cause inflammation of the thyroid gland, leading to thyroiditis.

5. Radiation Therapy: Exposure to radiation, particularly in the head and neck area, can lead to inflammation of the thyroid gland and thyroiditis.

Symptoms of Thyroiditis

The symptoms of thyroiditis can vary depending on the type and severity of inflammation. Common symptoms may include:

- Fatigue
- Weight gain or weight loss
- Sensitivity to cold or heat
- Muscle weakness
- Joint pain
- Depression or anxiety
- Dry skin and hair
- Brittle nails
- Irregular menstrual periods
- Difficulty concentrating
- Swelling in the neck (goiter)

In some cases, thyroiditis can cause hyperthyroidism (due to the release of excess thyroid hormones during inflammation) followed by hypothyroidism (as the thyroid gland becomes damaged and unable to produce enough hormones).

Diagnosis of Thyroiditis

The diagnosis of thyroiditis involves a combination of clinical evaluation, thyroid function tests, imaging studies, and sometimes biopsy. Key steps in the diagnostic process include:

1. Thyroid Function Tests: Blood tests are used to measure levels of thyroid hormones (T4 and T3) and thyroid-stimulating hormone (TSH). In thyroiditis, these levels can vary depending on the stage and type of inflammation. Early in the disease, there may be elevated levels of thyroid hormones due to inflammation, leading to hyperthyroidism. As the thyroid gland becomes damaged, hormone levels may decrease, resulting in hypothyroidism.

2. Thyroid Antibody Tests: In cases where autoimmune thyroiditis is suspected, antibody tests may be

performed to check for elevated levels of thyroid peroxidase antibodies (TPOAb) or thyroglobulin antibodies (TgAb). These antibodies are indicative of autoimmune thyroid disease.

3. Imaging Studies: Ultrasound may be used to assess the size, shape, and texture of the thyroid gland and to look for signs of inflammation or nodules. In some cases, a thyroid scan may be performed to evaluate the function of the thyroid gland.

4. Biopsy: In cases where a nodule or mass is present in the thyroid gland, a fine-needle aspiration biopsy (FNAB) may be performed to determine if it is cancerous or benign.

Treatment Approaches for Thyroiditis

The treatment of thyroiditis depends on the underlying cause and the specific type of thyroiditis. Treatment approaches may vary and can include:

1. Medications: Depending on the type of thyroiditis, your healthcare provider may prescribe medications to manage symptoms or to address the underlying cause:

   - Anti-inflammatory Medications: In cases of subacute thyroiditis or Hashimoto's thyroiditis, nonsteroidal anti-inflammatory drugs (NSAIDs) such as ibuprofen or aspirin may be used to reduce pain and inflammation.

   - Steroids: For more severe cases of subacute thyroiditis or Hashimoto's thyroiditis, corticosteroids such as prednisone may be prescribed to reduce inflammation and suppress the immune response against the thyroid gland.

   - Beta-Blockers: These medications, such as propranolol or atenolol, may be used to manage symptoms of hyperthyroidism in cases of subacute thyroiditis or to alleviate symptoms such as palpitations, tremors, and anxiety.

2. Hormone Replacement Therapy: In cases of hypothyroidism resulting from Hashimoto's thyroiditis, the mainstay of treatment is thyroid hormone replacement therapy with levothyroxine. This medication helps restore thyroid hormone levels to normal and alleviates symptoms of hypothyroidism. The dosage is adjusted based on thyroid function tests and symptoms.

3. Observation: In some cases, such as mild or transient forms of thyroiditis, no specific treatment may be needed other than close observation and monitoring of symptoms. Some types of thyroiditis, such as postpartum thyroiditis, may resolve on their own without the need for intervention.

4. Radioactive Iodine Therapy (RAI): In cases of silent or painless thyroiditis, which can sometimes result in transient hyperthyroidism followed by hypothyroidism, no specific treatment is usually required. However, if the hypothyroidism persists, thyroid hormone replacement therapy may be necessary.

5. Avoidance of Iodine: In cases of iodine-induced thyroiditis, such as amiodarone-induced thyroiditis, avoiding further exposure to iodine-containing substances is important to prevent exacerbation of thyroid dysfunction. This may involve discontinuing or reducing the dose of medications containing iodine.

6. Management of Complications: In rare cases, thyroiditis can lead to complications such as thyroid storm (severe hyperthyroidism), which requires immediate medical attention and intensive care

management. Treatment may include medications to control symptoms, supportive care, and, in severe cases, plasmapheresis or thyroidectomy.

Chapter 8: Thyroid and

Pregnancy

Importance of Thyroid Function During Pregnancy

Thyroid function plays a crucial role in pregnancy, as thyroid hormones are essential for the development of the fetus and the maintenance of a healthy pregnancy. The thyroid gland undergoes significant changes during pregnancy to meet the increased demand for thyroid hormones. Here are key aspects of the importance of thyroid function during pregnancy:

1. Fetal Brain Development: Thyroid hormones, particularly thyroxine (T4), are critical for the development of the fetal brain and nervous system. During the first trimester, before the fetal thyroid gland becomes functional, the fetus relies entirely on maternal thyroid hormones for proper brain development.

2. Metabolic Regulation: Thyroid hormones regulate metabolism in both the mother and the fetus, influencing energy production, growth, and development. Proper thyroid function is essential for maintaining normal metabolic processes during pregnancy.

3. Placental Function: Thyroid hormones play a role in the development and function of the placenta, which is crucial for providing nutrients and oxygen to the fetus and removing waste products.

4. Cardiovascular Health: Thyroid hormones are involved in regulating heart rate and cardiovascular function. Maintaining proper thyroid function is important for the cardiovascular health of both the mother and the fetus.

5. Growth and Development: Thyroid hormones contribute to the growth and development of various organs and tissues in the fetus, including the skeleton, muscles, and organs.

6. Regulation of Hormones: Thyroid hormones interact with other hormones, such as estrogen and

progesterone, which are important for maintaining pregnancy and preparing the body for childbirth.

7. Prevention of Complications: Proper thyroid function during pregnancy is associated with a lower risk of complications such as miscarriage, preterm birth, low birth weight, and developmental abnormalities.

Thyroid Function Tests During Pregnancy

During pregnancy, thyroid function is closely monitored to ensure that thyroid hormone levels remain within the normal range. The following tests are commonly used to assess thyroid function during pregnancy:

1. Thyroid-Stimulating Hormone (TSH): TSH is the most sensitive marker for thyroid function. During pregnancy, TSH levels naturally decrease due to the stimulatory effects of human chorionic gonadotropin (hCG), a hormone produced by the placenta. The reference range for TSH during pregnancy is lower than in non-pregnant individuals.

2. Free Thyroxine (FT4): FT4 levels are measured to assess the actual circulating levels of thyroxine (T4), the main thyroid hormone. FT4 levels should be maintained within the normal range to ensure proper thyroid function.

3. Thyroid Antibodies: Thyroid antibody tests, such as thyroid peroxidase antibodies (TPOAb) and thyroglobulin antibodies (TgAb), may be performed to screen for autoimmune thyroid disorders, such as Hashimoto's thyroiditis or Graves' disease, which can affect thyroid function during pregnancy.

4. Ultrasound Imaging: In some cases, thyroid ultrasound may be performed to assess the size, structure, and presence of nodules in the thyroid gland.

Management of Thyroid Disorders During Pregnancy

If thyroid dysfunction is detected during pregnancy, it is important to manage it promptly to ensure the health of both the mother and the fetus. Treatment approaches may include:

1. Thyroid Hormone Replacement: In cases of hypothyroidism, thyroid hormone replacement therapy with levothyroxine is usually prescribed to maintain normal thyroid hormone levels. The dosage may need to be adjusted during pregnancy to meet the increased demand for thyroid hormones.

2. Monitoring and Adjustments: Regular monitoring of thyroid function tests is essential during pregnancy to ensure that thyroid hormone levels remain within the normal range. The dosage of thyroid hormone replacement therapy may need to be adjusted based on these tests.

3. Management of Hyperthyroidism: In cases of hyperthyroidism, treatment options may include antithyroid medications to control thyroid hormone levels. Radioactive iodine therapy and thyroidectomy are generally avoided during pregnancy due to their potential effects on the fetus.

4. Collaboration with Healthcare Providers: Pregnant women with thyroid disorders should work closely with their healthcare providers, including obstetricians and endocrinologists, to ensure optimal management of their condition throughout pregnancy. This may

involve regular prenatal care visits and coordination of care between different specialists.

5. Postpartum Monitoring: Thyroid function should be reassessed after childbirth, as thyroid disorders can sometimes worsen or improve after pregnancy. Postpartum thyroiditis is a common condition characterized by transient hyperthyroidism followed by hypothyroidism, which may require monitoring and treatment.

Effects of Thyroid Disorders on Pregnancy and Fetal Development

Thyroid disorders can have significant implications for pregnancy and fetal development. The thyroid gland plays a crucial role in regulating metabolism and hormone production, which are essential for the proper development of the fetus. Here are the effects of various thyroid disorders on pregnancy and fetal development:

1. Hypothyroidism:
   - Impact on Pregnancy: Untreated or inadequately treated hypothyroidism during pregnancy can lead to complications such as miscarriage, preeclampsia (high

blood pressure during pregnancy), preterm birth, and low birth weight.

  - Fetal Development: Hypothyroidism can affect the development of the fetus, leading to cognitive impairments, developmental delays, and lower IQ scores in children born to mothers with untreated hypothyroidism.

2. Hyperthyroidism:

  - Impact on Pregnancy: Uncontrolled hyperthyroidism during pregnancy can increase the risk of miscarriage, preeclampsia, premature birth, and low birth weight. It can also lead to maternal heart failure or thyroid storm, a life-threatening condition.

  - Fetal Development: Hyperthyroidism can affect fetal development, leading to intrauterine growth restriction (IUGR), fetal tachycardia (rapid heartbeat), and in severe cases, fetal thyroid dysfunction.

3. Thyroid Nodules and Thyroid Cancer:

  - Impact on Pregnancy: Thyroid nodules and thyroid cancer are less common but can still impact pregnancy. Depending on the size and location of the nodules or cancer, they may require careful monitoring or treatment during pregnancy to prevent complications.

- Fetal Development: In cases where thyroid nodules or cancer require treatment during pregnancy, careful management is necessary to minimize the impact on fetal development. Radiation therapy and certain medications used to treat thyroid cancer are not safe during pregnancy and may need to be postponed until after delivery.

4. Postpartum Thyroiditis:
   - Impact on Pregnancy: Postpartum thyroiditis, characterized by transient hyperthyroidism followed by hypothyroidism, can occur in the first year after childbirth. It may lead to temporary thyroid dysfunction but usually resolves on its own without long-term consequences for future pregnancies.
   - Fetal Development: The effects of postpartum thyroiditis on fetal development are minimal, as the condition typically resolves before the next pregnancy.

5. Autoimmune Thyroid Disorders (Hashimoto's Thyroiditis, Graves' Disease):
   - Impact on Pregnancy: Women with autoimmune thyroid disorders are at an increased risk of infertility, miscarriage, and pregnancy complications such as preeclampsia and premature birth. Proper

management of these conditions before and during pregnancy is crucial to reduce these risks.

  - Fetal Development: Autoimmune thyroid disorders can affect fetal development, especially if thyroid hormone levels are not well-controlled. Adequate thyroid hormone replacement therapy or antithyroid medications may be necessary to ensure optimal fetal growth and development.

Management of Thyroid Disorders During Pregnancy

Thyroid disorders can have significant implications for pregnancy and fetal development. Proper management is crucial to ensure the health of both the mother and the baby. The management of thyroid disorders during pregnancy involves several key aspects:

1. Preconception Counseling: For women with known thyroid disorders who are planning to become pregnant, preconception counseling is important. This involves discussing the potential impact of thyroid disorders on pregnancy and the need for thyroid function tests before conception. Optimizing thyroid hormone levels before pregnancy can help reduce the risk of complications.

2. Thyroid Function Testing: Thyroid function tests, including TSH and free thyroxine (FT4) levels, should be monitored regularly during pregnancy. The target TSH range is lower during pregnancy than in non-pregnant individuals, typically between 0.1 and 2.5 mU/L in the first trimester and between 0.2 and 3.0 mU/L in the second and third trimesters. FT4 levels should be maintained within the normal range for pregnancy.

3. Thyroid Hormone Replacement Therapy: Women with hypothyroidism who are already on thyroid hormone replacement therapy should continue their medication during pregnancy. The dosage may need to be adjusted based on thyroid function tests. Levothyroxine is the preferred medication for hypothyroidism during pregnancy, as it is safe and effective for both the mother and the baby.

4. Monitoring and Adjustment of Medication: Thyroid function should be monitored approximately every 4-6 weeks during the first half of pregnancy and then at least once during the second half. The dosage of thyroid hormone replacement may need to be

adjusted to maintain thyroid function within the target range.

5. Management of Hyperthyroidism: Pregnant women with hyperthyroidism should be carefully monitored and treated to avoid complications such as preterm birth, low birth weight, and preeclampsia. Treatment options may include antithyroid medications (such as propylthiouracil or methimazole) to control thyroid hormone levels. These medications should be used at the lowest effective dose to minimize the risk of adverse effects on the baby.

6. Management of Thyroid Nodules and Cancer: Thyroid nodules detected during pregnancy should be evaluated with ultrasound and fine-needle aspiration biopsy if necessary. Treatment decisions depend on the size, characteristics, and risk of malignancy of the nodules. Thyroid cancer diagnosed during pregnancy may require surgical treatment or radioactive iodine therapy, with careful consideration of the potential risks to the fetus.

7. Iodine Supplementation: Adequate iodine intake is important for thyroid health during pregnancy. Pregnant women should consume iodine-rich foods or

take iodine supplements as recommended by their healthcare provider. Excessive iodine intake should be avoided, as it can also have negative effects on thyroid function.

8. Postpartum Monitoring: Thyroid function should be re-evaluated after delivery, as thyroid hormone requirements may change. Some women with autoimmune thyroiditis may develop postpartum thyroiditis, characterized by transient hyperthyroidism followed by hypothyroidism. Close monitoring and appropriate management are essential during this period.

9. Collaborative Care: Managing thyroid disorders during pregnancy often requires collaboration between obstetricians, endocrinologists, and other healthcare providers. This multidisciplinary approach helps ensure comprehensive care that addresses both maternal and fetal health.

10. Education and Support: Pregnant women with thyroid disorders should receive education about their condition, treatment options, and the importance of adherence to medication and follow-up appointments. Supportive care from healthcare providers and

support groups can also be beneficial in managing the challenges of pregnancy with a thyroid disorder.

Chapter 9: Thyroid Eye Disease

(Graves' Ophthalmopathy)

Causes and Risk Factors

Thyroid eye disease (TED), also known as Graves' ophthalmopathy, is an autoimmune condition that primarily affects the tissues around the eyes. The exact cause of TED is not fully understood, but it is believed to involve a combination of genetic, environmental, and immune system factors. The following are key factors thought to contribute to the development of TED:

1. Autoimmune Reaction: TED is often associated with Graves' disease, an autoimmune disorder characterized by an overactive thyroid gland (hyperthyroidism). In Graves' disease, the immune system mistakenly attacks the thyroid gland, leading to excessive production of thyroid hormones. It is

believed that the same autoimmune process can also affect the tissues around the eyes, leading to TED. The exact mechanisms by which this autoimmune reaction occurs are not fully understood.

2. Thyroid-Stimulating Hormone Receptor (TSH-R) Antibodies: In Graves' disease and TED, the immune system produces antibodies that target the thyroid-stimulating hormone receptor (TSH-R) on the surface of thyroid cells. These antibodies can also bind to TSH-R on the cells of the orbital tissues around the eyes, leading to inflammation and tissue damage. This process is thought to play a key role in the development of TED.

3. Genetic Predisposition: There is evidence to suggest that genetic factors may contribute to the development of TED. Certain genetic variations may increase the susceptibility to autoimmune conditions, including Graves' disease and TED. However, the specific genes involved and their exact roles in TED are still being studied.

4. Environmental Triggers: Environmental factors, such as smoking, stress, and infections, may trigger or exacerbate the autoimmune response in TED. Smoking,

in particular, is a significant risk factor for the development and severity of TED. It is believed to worsen inflammation and contribute to tissue damage in the eyes.

5. Female Gender: TED is more common in women than in men, with a female-to-male ratio of approximately 5:1. The reason for this gender difference is not fully understood but may be related to hormonal factors or differences in the immune response between men and women.

6. Age and Disease Severity: TED typically occurs in middle-aged adults, with the peak incidence between the ages of 30 and 50. The severity of TED can vary widely, ranging from mild eye symptoms to severe and sight-threatening complications. The risk of developing TED is higher in individuals with more severe Graves' disease.

7. Other Autoimmune Conditions: People with TED may have other autoimmune conditions, such as rheumatoid arthritis, lupus, or type 1 diabetes. The presence of multiple autoimmune conditions suggests a generalized dysregulation of the immune system.

While these factors are believed to contribute to the development of TED, the exact interplay between genetic, environmental, and immune factors in triggering the disease is complex and not fully understood. Further research is needed to elucidate the underlying mechanisms and to develop more effective treatments for TED.

Symptoms of Thyroid Eye Disease

Thyroid eye disease, also known as Graves' ophthalmopathy, is an autoimmune condition that affects the eyes and is often associated with Graves' disease, an autoimmune disorder that affects the thyroid gland. The symptoms of thyroid eye disease can vary in severity and may include:

1. Eye Bulging (Proptosis): One of the most characteristic features of thyroid eye disease is the protrusion of one or both eyes, known as proptosis or exophthalmos. This occurs due to inflammation and swelling of the tissues behind the eyes, which pushes the eyeballs forward. Proptosis can cause a prominent or "staring" appearance and may lead to exposure of the cornea, making the eyes more vulnerable to irritation and dryness.

2. Double Vision (Diplopia): Thyroid eye disease can affect the alignment of the eyes, leading to double vision or diplopia. This occurs when the muscles that control eye movement become inflamed and weakened, causing the eyes to not move together properly. Double vision can be constant or intermittent and may worsen with certain eye movements or positions.

3. Eye Pain: Inflammation of the tissues around the eyes can cause eye pain, which may be described as aching, sharp, or stabbing. The pain may worsen with eye movement or when the eyes are exposed to bright light. Eye pain can also be associated with headaches and discomfort around the temples or forehead.

4. Swelling and Redness: The eyelids and the tissues around the eyes may become swollen and red due to inflammation. This can contribute to the appearance of bulging eyes and may be accompanied by a feeling of pressure or fullness around the eyes.

5. Dryness and Irritation: Thyroid eye disease can lead to dryness, irritation, and a gritty sensation in the eyes. This is often due to decreased tear production or poor

distribution of tears over the surface of the eyes, resulting from changes in the eyelids' position and the exposure of the cornea.

6. Difficulty Closing the Eyes: In severe cases, the swelling and inflammation around the eyes can affect the ability to fully close the eyelids, leading to exposure of the cornea during sleep (lagophthalmos). This can increase the risk of corneal abrasions and infections.

7. Changes in Vision: Some people with thyroid eye disease may experience changes in vision, such as blurred vision, decreased visual acuity, or sensitivity to light (photophobia). These changes can be due to corneal exposure, optic nerve compression, or other effects of the disease on the eyes.

It's important to note that not all individuals with thyroid eye disease will experience all of these symptoms, and the severity of symptoms can vary widely. Some people may have mild symptoms that improve over time, while others may experience more severe and persistent symptoms that require medical intervention. Early recognition and treatment of thyroid eye disease are crucial to prevent complications and preserve vision.

Treatment Options for Thyroid Eye Disease

Thyroid eye disease (TED), also known as Graves' ophthalmopathy, is an autoimmune condition that affects the eyes and surrounding tissues. The goal of treatment is to manage symptoms, reduce inflammation, and prevent complications. Treatment options for TED may include:

1. Steroids: Oral or intravenous corticosteroids, such as prednisone, are commonly used to reduce inflammation in the eyes and surrounding tissues. Steroids can help alleviate symptoms such as eye pain, redness, swelling, and double vision. The dosage and duration of steroid treatment are determined based on the severity of symptoms and response to treatment. Steroid treatment may be tapered gradually to prevent rebound inflammation.

2. Orbital Decompression Surgery: In cases where TED causes severe eye bulging (proptosis) or compression of the optic nerve, orbital decompression surgery may be recommended. This surgical procedure involves

removing bone or fat from the eye socket to create more space for the swollen tissues. Orbital decompression can help improve eye appearance, reduce proptosis, and relieve pressure on the optic nerve, which is important for preserving vision.

3. Radiation Therapy: External beam radiation therapy (EBRT) or orbital radiotherapy may be considered for TED that is not responsive to other treatments or for patients who are not suitable candidates for surgery. Radiation therapy can help reduce inflammation and swelling in the eye tissues. It is usually reserved for severe or refractory cases of TED due to potential side effects and long-term risks.

4. Eye Lubrication and Protection: Lubricating eye drops or ointments can help relieve dryness and irritation associated with TED. Wearing sunglasses and using artificial tears can protect the eyes from exposure to wind, dust, and sunlight, which can exacerbate symptoms.

5. Prism Glasses: For patients with double vision (diplopia) caused by TED, prism glasses can help align the images seen by each eye, reducing the perception of double vision.

6. Thyroid Treatment: Managing the underlying thyroid dysfunction, such as hyperthyroidism in Graves' disease, is important in the overall management of TED. Controlling thyroid hormone levels with antithyroid medications, radioactive iodine therapy, or thyroidectomy can help stabilize TED symptoms.

7. Smoking Cessation: Smoking has been linked to the worsening of TED symptoms and can interfere with treatment outcomes. Quitting smoking is strongly recommended for patients with TED.

8. Regular Monitoring: Patients with TED require regular monitoring by an ophthalmologist to assess the progression of the disease, monitor for complications such as optic nerve compression, and adjust treatment as needed.

Chapter 10: Thyroid Diet and

Lifestyle

Foods to Support Thyroid Function

A healthy diet plays a crucial role in supporting thyroid function and overall well-being. While there is no specific "thyroid diet," incorporating certain nutrients and foods can help support thyroid health. Here are some foods that are beneficial for thyroid function:

1. Iodine-Rich Foods: Iodine is an essential mineral required for the production of thyroid hormones. Good sources of iodine include iodized salt, seaweed (such as kelp, nori, and wakame), seafood (such as fish, shrimp, and shellfish), dairy products, and eggs. However, excessive iodine intake can also be detrimental to thyroid health, so it's important to consume iodine in moderation.

2. Selenium: Selenium is another important mineral that is essential for thyroid function. It helps convert the inactive thyroid hormone T4 into the active form T3. Selenium-rich foods include Brazil nuts, seafood (such as tuna, sardines, and shrimp), eggs, sunflower seeds, and mushrooms.

3. Zinc: Zinc is involved in the synthesis of thyroid hormones and is important for immune function. Foods high in zinc include oysters, beef, chicken, nuts (such as cashews and almonds), seeds (such as pumpkin seeds and sesame seeds), and legumes (such as lentils and chickpeas).

4. Iron: Iron deficiency can affect thyroid function and lead to hypothyroidism. Iron-rich foods include red meat, poultry, fish, lentils, beans, spinach, and fortified cereals.

5. Vitamin D: Adequate vitamin D levels are important for thyroid health and immune function. Sources of vitamin D include sunlight exposure, fatty fish (such as salmon and mackerel), egg yolks, and fortified foods (such as milk, orange juice, and cereals).

6. Omega-3 Fatty Acids: Omega-3 fatty acids have anti-inflammatory properties and may help reduce inflammation in the thyroid gland. Sources of omega-3s include fatty fish (such as salmon, sardines, and mackerel), flaxseeds, chia seeds, walnuts, and soybeans.

7. Antioxidant-Rich Foods: Antioxidants help protect the thyroid gland from oxidative stress and inflammation. Foods rich in antioxidants include fruits (such as berries, citrus fruits, and grapes), vegetables (such as spinach, kale, and broccoli), nuts, seeds, and green tea.

8. Probiotic Foods: Probiotics may help support gut health, which is important for thyroid function and immune function. Fermented foods such as yogurt, kefir, kimchi, sauerkraut, and miso are good sources of probiotics.

It's important to maintain a balanced diet that includes a variety of nutrient-rich foods to support overall health and thyroid function. Avoiding excessive intake of processed foods, refined sugars, and unhealthy fats can also help maintain a healthy thyroid.

Lifestyle Factors Affecting Thyroid Health

In addition to dietary considerations, several lifestyle factors can impact thyroid health. Managing these factors can help support overall thyroid function and improve well-being. Key lifestyle factors affecting thyroid health include:

1. Stress Management: Chronic stress can negatively impact thyroid function by affecting hormone balance and immune function. Stress management techniques such as mindfulness meditation, yoga, deep breathing exercises, and regular physical activity can help reduce stress levels and support thyroid health.

2. Exercise: Regular physical activity is beneficial for thyroid health. Exercise can help improve metabolism, promote weight management, and reduce inflammation, which can be beneficial for individuals with thyroid disorders. Aim for a combination of aerobic exercises (such as walking, jogging, cycling) and strength training exercises (such as weightlifting, resistance band exercises) for overall health and fitness.

3. Sleep: Quality sleep is essential for overall health, including thyroid function. Poor sleep can disrupt hormone production and metabolism, leading to imbalances that may affect thyroid health. Aim for 7-9 hours of restful sleep per night and practice good sleep hygiene habits, such as maintaining a regular sleep schedule, creating a comfortable sleep environment, and avoiding stimulants like caffeine and electronics before bedtime.

4. Smoking Cessation: Smoking has been linked to an increased risk of thyroid disorders, including Graves' disease and thyroid cancer. Quitting smoking can improve thyroid function and overall health. Seek support from healthcare providers or smoking cessation programs if you need help quitting.

5. Alcohol Consumption: Excessive alcohol consumption can interfere with thyroid hormone production and metabolism. Limiting alcohol intake to moderate levels (up to one drink per day for women and up to two drinks per day for men) is recommended for overall health and thyroid function.

6. Environmental Factors: Environmental toxins and pollutants, such as heavy metals (e.g., mercury, lead),

pesticides, and industrial chemicals, can affect thyroid function. Minimize exposure to these toxins by choosing organic foods, using natural cleaning products, and avoiding products containing harmful chemicals.

7. Nutrient Deficiencies: Certain nutrients are essential for thyroid function, including iodine, selenium, zinc, iron, and vitamins A, D, and B12. A balanced diet that includes a variety of nutrient-dense foods can help prevent deficiencies. If you have specific nutrient deficiencies, your healthcare provider may recommend supplements to address them.

8. Hydration: Adequate hydration is important for overall health and can support thyroid function. Aim to drink enough water throughout the day to stay hydrated.

Appendix

Stress Management Techniques

Relaxation Techniques: Meditation, Breathing Exercises, Yoga and Tai Chi

Stress management is an essential aspect of healthy living, as stress can exacerbate illnesses and impact overall well-being. Incorporating relaxation techniques into daily life can help individuals with any chronic condition reduce stress levels and improve their ability to cope with the challenges of their condition. Two effective relaxation techniques are meditation and breathing exercises:

1. Meditation:
   - Meditation is a practice that involves focusing the mind and eliminating distractions to achieve a state of relaxation and mental clarity.
   - Guided meditation, mindfulness meditation, and mantra meditation are popular techniques that can be

practiced individually or with the help of audio guides or apps.

Techniques
- • Guided Meditation
- Find a quiet and comfortable place where you can sit or lie down without distractions.
- Close your eyes and take a few deep breaths to relax your body and mind.
- Start the guided meditation recording or app of your choice.
- Follow the instructions of the guide, which may involve visualizations, breathing exercises, or body scans.
- Focus on the guide's voice and the instructions, allowing yourself to let go of any thoughts or distractions.
- Continue to follow the guide's instructions until the meditation session is complete.
- Take a few moments to rest and notice how you feel before returning to your usual activities.

- • Mindfulness Meditation
- Find a comfortable seated position with your back straight but relaxed.

- Close your eyes or gaze softly at a spot in front of you.
- Begin by bringing your attention to your breath, noticing the sensation of the breath as it enters and leaves your body.
- As thoughts, sensations, or emotions arise, acknowledge them without judgment and gently bring your focus back to your breath.
- Continue to observe your breath, returning to it whenever your mind wanders.
- Practice this for a predetermined amount of time, such as 5 or 10 minutes, gradually increasing the duration as you become more comfortable with the practice.
- When you're ready, slowly open your eyes and take a moment to transition back to your surroundings.

- Mantra Meditation
- Choose a word, phrase, or sound (mantra) that resonates with you and has positive associations.
- Find a comfortable seated position with your back straight but relaxed.
- Close your eyes and take a few deep breaths to center yourself.

- Begin silently repeating your chosen mantra with each breath, focusing on the sound or feeling of the mantra.

- If your mind wanders, gently bring your focus back to the mantra without judgment.

- Continue to repeat the mantra for a predetermined amount of time, such as 5 or 10 minutes.

- When you're ready, slowly release the mantra and take a few moments to rest before returning to your usual activities.

2. Breathing Exercises

- Breathing exercises, also known as deep breathing or diaphragmatic breathing, can help calm the mind and body by promoting relaxation and reducing the body's stress response.

- To practice deep breathing, individuals should find a comfortable position and focus on taking slow, deep breaths in through the nose, filling the abdomen with air, and then exhaling slowly through the mouth.

- Deep breathing can be practiced anywhere and anytime, making it a convenient and accessible stress management technique.

Technique

- Find a Comfortable Position
    - Sit or lie down in a comfortable position, with your back straight but relaxed. You can also practice deep breathing while standing if that's more comfortable for you.

- Relax Your Body
    - Close your eyes if you're comfortable doing so, and take a few moments to relax your body. Release any tension in your muscles, starting from your head and working down to your toes.

- Focus on Your Breath
    - Begin to pay attention to your breath without trying to control it. Notice the natural rhythm of your breathing, the rise and fall of your chest or abdomen with each breath.

- Inhale Slowly Through Your Nose
    - Take a slow, deep breath in through your nose, allowing your abdomen to expand as you fill your lungs with air. Try to

> inhale for a count of 4 or 5 seconds, or whatever feels comfortable for you.

- Exhale Slowly Through Your Mouth
  - Exhale slowly and completely through your mouth, allowing your abdomen to contract as you release the air from your lungs. Try to exhale for a count of 4 or 5 seconds, or whatever feels comfortable for you.

- Repeat
  - Continue this slow, deep breathing pattern, focusing on the sensation of your breath as it enters and leaves your body. Inhale deeply, exhale completely, and pause briefly before the next breath.

- Counting Your Breaths
  - If it helps you focus, you can count your breaths. For example, count silently to yourself as you inhale (1, 2, 3, 4), hold your breath for a moment, and then count as you exhale (1, 2, 3, 4).

- Practice for Several Minutes

- Practice deep breathing for several minutes, gradually increasing the duration as you become more comfortable with the technique. Aim for 5 to 10 minutes initially, and you can extend the duration as you feel more at ease.

- Transition Back to Normal Breathing
  - When you're ready to finish, take a few normal breaths and gradually return to your regular breathing pattern. Notice how you feel after practicing deep breathing.

- Practice Regularly
  - To experience the benefits of deep breathing, practice this technique regularly. You can incorporate deep breathing into your daily routine, such as before bedtime or during moments of stress or anxiety.

3. Tai Chi Exercises:

- "Cloud Hands" (Yun Shou):

- Start in a relaxed standing position with your feet shoulder-width apart and your knees slightly bent.
- Begin by shifting your weight to your right leg and turning your torso to the right, allowing your arms to follow in a circular motion.
- As you shift your weight to your left leg, continue the circular motion of your arms to the left.
- Repeat this flowing motion, coordinating the movement of your arms with the shifting of your weight from one leg to the other.
- Focus on maintaining a relaxed and flowing rhythm throughout the exercise.

- "Repulse Monkey" (Dao Nian Hou):
- Begin in a standing position with your feet shoulder-width apart and your knees slightly bent.
- Shift your weight to your right leg and step back with your left foot, keeping your toes pointed slightly outward.
- As you step back, turn your torso to the left and extend your arms in front of you, palms facing outward.
- Shift your weight back to your left leg, bringing your right foot back to the starting position.
- Repeat this sequence, alternating sides with each repetition.

- Focus on maintaining a smooth and controlled movement, coordinating the stepping and arm movements.

- "Grasp the Sparrow's Tail" (Lan Que Wei):
- Begin in a standing position with your feet shoulder-width apart and your knees slightly bent.
- Start with your arms relaxed at your sides.
- Shift your weight to your right leg and step back with your left foot, keeping your toes pointed slightly outward.
- As you step back, turn your torso to the left and extend your arms in front of you, palms facing outward.
- Shift your weight back to your left leg, bringing your right foot back to the starting position.
- Repeat this sequence, alternating sides with each repetition.
- Focus on maintaining a smooth and controlled movement, coordinating the stepping and arm movements.

4. Yoga Exercises:

- Tree Pose (Vrikshasana):

- Begin in a standing position with your feet together and your arms at your sides.
- Shift your weight onto your left foot and lift your right foot off the ground.
- Place the sole of your right foot on the inner left thigh or calf, avoiding the knee joint.
- Press your foot into your leg and your leg into your foot to create a stable base.
- Bring your palms together in front of your chest in a prayer position, or raise your arms overhead.
- Hold the pose for 30 seconds to 1 minute, then switch sides.

- Warrior III Pose (Virabhadrasana III):
- Begin in a standing position with your feet hip-width apart and your arms at your sides.
- Shift your weight onto your left foot and lift your right foot off the ground.
- Hinge forward at the hips, extending your right leg behind you and reaching your arms forward.
- Keep your hips and shoulders square to the ground, and your body forming a straight line from head to heel.
- Hold the pose for 30 seconds to 1 minute, then switch sides.

- Half Moon Pose (Ardha Chandrasana):
  - Begin in a standing position with your feet together and your arms at your sides.
  - Step your left foot back about 3-4 feet and turn your left foot out about 45 degrees.
  - Extend your arms out to the sides at shoulder height.
  - Shift your weight onto your right foot and lift your left leg off the ground.
  - Rotate your torso to the left and bring your left arm down to the floor, either inside or outside of your right foot.
  - Extend your right arm toward the ceiling, creating a "half moon" shape with your body.
  - Hold the pose for 30 seconds to 1 minute, then switch sides.

Resources for Further Information

and Support

Managing a thyroid disorder can be challenging, but there are many resources available to provide information, support, and guidance. Here are some resources you may find helpful:

1. Healthcare Providers: Your primary care physician, endocrinologist, or other healthcare providers are valuable sources of information and support. They can provide personalized advice, treatment options, and referrals to specialists if needed. Regular check-ups and open communication with your healthcare team are important for managing your thyroid condition effectively.

2. Thyroid Organizations and Websites: There are several reputable organizations and websites dedicated to thyroid health that offer reliable information, educational materials, and support networks. Some of these include:

- American Thyroid Association (ATA): Provides comprehensive information on thyroid disorders, treatment options, and research updates. Their website offers patient resources, educational materials, and a directory of healthcare providers.
- Thyroid Foundation of Canada: Offers educational resources, support groups, and advocacy initiatives for individuals with thyroid disorders in Canada.
- British Thyroid Foundation: Provides information, support, and resources for people with thyroid disorders in the UK, including educational materials and a helpline.
- Thyroid Federation International: A global network of thyroid patient organizations that offers resources, support, and advocacy efforts for thyroid patients worldwide.

3. Online Communities and Support Groups: Joining online communities and support groups can connect you with others who have similar experiences with thyroid disorders. These groups can provide a sense of community, emotional support, and practical tips for managing your condition. Websites like Inspire, Thyroid UK, and Thyroid Support Group (on Facebook) are popular platforms for connecting with others affected by thyroid disorders.

4. Books and Publications: There are many books and publications available that provide in-depth information on thyroid health, including diagnosis, treatment options, and lifestyle management. Some recommended books include "Thyroid for Dummies" by Alan L. Rubin, MD, and "The Thyroid Connection" by Amy Myers, MD.

5. Patient Advocacy Groups: Organizations such as the Thyroid Cancer Survivors' Association (ThyCa) and ThyroidChange advocate for thyroid patients' rights, raise awareness about thyroid disorders, and provide support and resources for patients and caregivers.

6. Educational Events and Webinars: Keep an eye out for educational events, webinars, and conferences focused on thyroid health. These events often feature expert speakers who provide up-to-date information on thyroid disorders, treatment advancements, and lifestyle management strategies.

Explanation of Common Thyroid Function Tests

Thyroid function tests are blood tests used to assess the function of the thyroid gland and the levels of thyroid hormones in the body. These tests are essential for diagnosing thyroid disorders, monitoring treatment effectiveness, and guiding medication adjustments. The most common thyroid function tests include:

1. Thyroid-Stimulating Hormone (TSH): TSH is produced by the pituitary gland in response to the levels of thyroid hormones (T3 and T4) in the bloodstream. High TSH levels indicate an underactive thyroid (hypothyroidism), as the pituitary gland tries to stimulate the thyroid to produce more hormones. Low TSH levels suggest an overactive thyroid (hyperthyroidism), as the pituitary gland reduces TSH production to suppress thyroid hormone production.

   - Reference Range: The normal reference range for TSH levels can vary slightly depending on the laboratory and the specific assay used. In general, the reference range for TSH is between 0.4 and 4.0 milliunits per liter (mU/L). However, some experts suggest that the upper limit of the normal range should be lower, around 2.5 mU/L, especially for individuals without thyroid disease symptoms.

2. Free Thyroxine (FT4): FT4 is the active form of thyroid hormone that is not bound to proteins in the blood. It represents the amount of thyroid hormone available for use by the body's tissues. Low FT4 levels indicate hypothyroidism, while high FT4 levels suggest hyperthyroidism.

   - Reference Range: The normal reference range for FT4 levels is typically between 0.8 and 1.8 nanograms per deciliter (ng/dL).

3. Total Thyroxine (T4): Total T4 includes both free T4 and T4 that is bound to proteins in the blood. This test is less commonly used than FT4 but can provide additional information about thyroid function.

   - Reference Range: The normal reference range for total T4 levels is approximately 4.5 to 12.5 micrograms per deciliter (mcg/dL).

4. Free Triiodothyronine (FT3): FT3 is the active form of thyroid hormone that is not bound to proteins in the blood. It is a less commonly ordered test than FT4 but can provide additional insights into thyroid function, especially in cases of suspected hyperthyroidism or thyroid hormone resistance.

   - Reference Range: The normal reference range for FT3 levels is typically between 2.3 and 4.2 picograms per milliliter (pg/mL).

5. Thyroid Antibodies: Thyroid antibodies are proteins produced by the immune system that can attack the thyroid gland, leading to autoimmune thyroid disorders such as Hashimoto's thyroiditis and Graves' disease. The two main types of thyroid antibodies tested are thyroid peroxidase antibodies (TPOAb) and thyroglobulin antibodies (TgAb).

   - Reference Range: The presence of thyroid antibodies is indicative of autoimmune thyroid disease. Reference ranges for specific antibody levels may vary depending on the laboratory and the assay used.

Glossary

1. Thyroid Gland: A butterfly-shaped gland located in the front of the neck, responsible for producing hormones that regulate metabolism, growth, and development.

2. Thyroid Hormones: Hormones produced by the thyroid gland, including thyroxine (T4) and triiodothyronine (T3), which play a key role in regulating metabolism, heart rate, and body temperature.

3. Thyroid Stimulating Hormone (TSH): A hormone produced by the pituitary gland that stimulates the thyroid gland to produce T4 and T3.

4. Hyperthyroidism: A condition where the thyroid gland is overactive and produces excessive amounts of thyroid hormones, leading to symptoms such as weight loss, rapid heart rate, and anxiety.

5. Hypothyroidism: A condition where the thyroid gland is underactive and does not produce enough

thyroid hormones, leading to symptoms such as fatigue, weight gain, and depression.

6. Goiter: An enlarged thyroid gland, often caused by iodine deficiency or thyroid disorders such as hyperthyroidism or hypothyroidism.

7. Graves' Disease: An autoimmune disorder that causes hyperthyroidism, characterized by the production of antibodies that stimulate the thyroid gland to produce excessive thyroid hormones.

8. Hashimoto's Thyroiditis: An autoimmune disorder that causes hypothyroidism, characterized by inflammation of the thyroid gland and the production of antibodies that attack the thyroid tissue.

9. Thyroid Nodule: A small abnormal growth or lump in the thyroid gland, which may be benign (non-cancerous) or malignant (cancerous).

10. Thyroid Cancer: Cancer that develops in the cells of the thyroid gland, which can be classified as papillary, follicular, medullary, or anaplastic thyroid cancer.

11. Thyroidectomy: Surgical removal of part or all of the thyroid gland, often performed to treat thyroid cancer, goiter, or hyperthyroidism.

12. Radioactive Iodine Therapy: A treatment for hyperthyroidism or thyroid cancer that involves the oral administration of radioactive iodine, which is taken up by the thyroid gland and destroys thyroid tissue.

13. Thyroid Storm: A life-threatening complication of untreated or poorly managed hyperthyroidism, characterized by severe symptoms such as high fever, rapid heart rate, and confusion.

14. Thyroid Eye Disease: Also known as Graves' ophthalmopathy, a condition associated with Graves' disease characterized by eye symptoms such as bulging eyes (exophthalmos), double vision, and eye irritation.

15. Thyroid Function Tests: Blood tests used to assess thyroid function, including TSH, free T4, total T3, free T3, TPO antibodies, and thyroglobulin antibodies.

16. Subclinical Hyperthyroidism: A condition where TSH levels are low but thyroid hormone levels (T4 and T3) are within the normal range, often without obvious symptoms.

17. Subclinical Hypothyroidism: A condition where TSH levels are high but thyroid hormone levels (T4 and T3) are within the normal range, often without obvious symptoms.

18. Thyroiditis: Inflammation of the thyroid gland, which can be caused by infections, autoimmune disorders, or other factors.

19. Thyroid Ultrasound: A non-invasive imaging test that uses sound waves to create images of the thyroid gland, often used to evaluate thyroid nodules or thyroid size.

20. Thyroid Fine Needle Aspiration (FNA) Biopsy: A procedure used to collect cells from thyroid nodules for examination under a microscope to determine if the nodule is benign or malignant.

21. Thyroid Hormone Resistance: A rare condition where the body's tissues are resistant to the effects of

thyroid hormones, despite normal or elevated levels of thyroid hormones in the blood.

22. Thyroid Binding Globulin (TBG): A protein produced by the liver that binds to thyroid hormones in the blood, regulating their transport and availability to tissues.

23. Thyroid Hormone Replacement Therapy: Treatment for hypothyroidism that involves taking synthetic thyroid hormones (levothyroxine) to replace the hormones not produced by the thyroid gland.

24. Euthyroid: A state where thyroid function is normal, with normal levels of TSH and thyroid hormones.

25. Thyroid Storm: A life-threatening complication of untreated or poorly managed hyperthyroidism, characterized by severe symptoms such as high fever, rapid heart rate, and confusion.

26. Thyroid Autoimmunity: An immune response where the body's immune system mistakenly attacks the thyroid gland, leading to autoimmune thyroid disorders such as Hashimoto's thyroiditis and Graves' disease.

27. Thyroid Hormone Transporters: Proteins that facilitate the transport of thyroid hormones across cell membranes, regulating their uptake and availability to tissues.

28. Thyroid Hormone Receptors: Proteins located on the surface of cells that bind to thyroid hormones, initiating cellular responses that regulate metabolism, growth, and development.

29. Thyroid Function in Pregnancy: Changes in thyroid function during pregnancy, including increased production of thyroid hormones to support fetal development, which can lead to temporary thyroid dysfunction in some women.

30. Postpartum Thyroiditis: Thyroid dysfunction that occurs in the first year after childbirth, characterized by temporary hyperthyroidism followed by hypothyroidism in some women.

31. Thyroid Hormone Regulation: The complex feedback mechanism involving the hypothalamus, pituitary gland, and thyroid gland that regulates the production and release of thyroid hormones.

32. Thyroid Hormone Signaling Pathways: Intracellular pathways that mediate the effects of thyroid hormones on gene expression and cellular functions.

33. Thyroid Hormone Metabolism: The process by which thyroid hormones are synthesized, transported, metabolized, and excreted by the body.

34. Thyroid Hormone Resistance Syndrome: A rare genetic disorder characterized by reduced responsiveness of tissues to thyroid hormones, leading to symptoms of hypothyroidism despite normal or elevated thyroid hormone levels in the blood.

35. Thyroid Hormone Synthesis: The process by which the thyroid gland produces thyroid hormones (T4 and T3) from iodine and the amino acid tyrosine.

36. Thyroid Hormone Feedback Mechanism: The mechanism by which levels of thyroid hormones in the blood regulate the secretion of TSH by the pituitary gland and TSH production by the hypothalamus.

37. Thyroid Hormone Transport Proteins: Proteins that bind to thyroid hormones in the blood, transporting them to target tissues and regulating their availability for cellular uptake.

38. Thyroid Hormone Receptor Mutations: Genetic mutations that affect the function of thyroid hormone receptors, leading to altered thyroid hormone signaling and metabolism.

39. Thyroid Hormone Resistance: A condition where tissues in the body are less responsive to thyroid hormones, leading to symptoms of hypothyroidism despite normal or elevated levels of thyroid hormones in the blood.

40. Thyroid Hormone Deficiency: A condition where the body does not produce enough thyroid hormones, leading to symptoms of hypothyroidism such as fatigue, weight gain, and cold intolerance.